Jhon Ypanaque
Dario Paquiyauri
José Luis Saly Rosas

Lifestyles of midwifery students

Jhon Ypanaque
Dario Paquiyauri
José Luis Saly Rosas

Lifestyles of midwifery students

Northern Peru

ScienciaScripts

Imprint
Any brand names and product names mentioned in this book are subject to trademark, brand or patent protection and are trademarks or registered trademarks of their respective holders. The use of brand names, product names, common names, trade names, product descriptions etc. even without a particular marking in this work is in no way to be construed to mean that such names may be regarded as unrestricted in respect of trademark and brand protection legislation and could thus be used by anyone.

Cover image: www.ingimage.com

This book is a translation from the original published under ISBN 978-620-3-03679-4.

Publisher:
Sciencia Scripts
is a trademark of
International Book Market Service Ltd., member of OmniScriptum Publishing Group
17 Meldrum Street, Beau Bassin 71504, Mauritius
Printed at: see last page
ISBN: 978-620-3-49250-7

CHAPTER I

INTRODUCTION

Within a society, health will always be considered as one of the most essential rights. It is defined as the complete state of physical, psychological and social well-being and not only the absence of illness, which aims to achieve an ever better quality of life and to constantly improve the social and individual conditions in which every human being lives. Thus, even the Peruvian laws within its political constitution refer to the protection of health.

It is known that there are currently different factors that modify the optimal state of health of human beings, which generate changes in their behaviour, preventing them from enjoying a good quality of life, such lifestyles give rise to different non-communicable diseases that are currently the new epidemic that is sweeping the world.

It is difficult to find human behaviours that do not influence health and well-being, which is why there are a number of scenarios where these are considered risk factors for major health problems. These currently include drinking alcoholic beverages, smoking tobacco, dietary imbalances, not engaging in physical activity, not taking part in health promotion activities, disregarding doctor's instructions and using health services inappropriately, among others [1].

The World Health Organisation (WHO) states that adolescents between 19 and 24 years of age is a period of life in which the individual prepares for work and for assuming adult life with all its responsibilities. The majority of university students are in their late adolescence [2].

Adolescence is a crucial time and both health and nutrition on university campuses lacked this preventive focus.

The university is not only a place where students can learn, but it is also a place where they are able to learn. At that time, university life was considered to take place solely within the confines of classrooms and libraries; however, it is now recognised that the performance of university students will depend to a large extent on their lifestyle, nutrition and both physical and mental health3.

In addition to this, it should be noted that during the university period, people learn behaviours that often last into adulthood. For this reason, activities that promote and prevent health problems are key for the population at this stage, as their lifestyles will have a direct influence on their mental, physical and mental development [2.]

This is where the importance of a good lifestyle lies in order to obtain positive results in the health and safety of both themselves and their patients in the future. Therefore, by evaluating the lifestyles of obstetricians in training, it will be possible to know aspects related to their health in order to be able to inform them of the related risks and make them aware of them, which is fundamental to improve the gear made up of prevention, care, and promotion of sexual and reproductive health.

The aforementioned motivated the author to approach this particular subject through the scientific method, formulating the question:
What are the lifestyles of the students of the School of Midwifery of the National University of Tumbes 2018?

Therefore, the general objective was set as a general objective:

To determine the lifestyles of the students of the School of Obstetrics of the Faculty of Health Sciences of the National University of Tumbes 2018. And as specific objectives:

1. Identify the physical activity that students do.
2. Identify students' eating habits.
3. Assess students' sleep and stress.
4. Identify students' consumption of toxic substances.

CHAPTER II

FRAME OF REFERENCE

2.1. BACKGROUND:

A review of studies on the subject has shown the importance of improving the lifestyle of students at the School of Midwifery, and we present below the main background information reported:

At the international level, Benassar[4] , in the descriptive study Lifestyles and health in university students at the University of Illes Balears in Spain in 2011, using Delphi methodology, found that 65.8% of students were physically active, 19.5% of students were smokers and 58% of students were alcohol consumers.

Trujillo and Wilman[5] , in their descriptive cross-sectional study, entitled Sleep and Time Allocation among students at the Universidad del Atlántico in Barranquilla (Colombia), surveyed students enrolled in undergraduate programmes in the first semester of 2009, where they concluded that the optimal choice of sleep for students at the Universidad del Atlántico is between 5.57 and 12 hours per day.

Ratner et al[6] , in their cross-sectional study conducted in Chile in 2012, analysed the dietary behaviour, nutritional status and disease history of 6,823 students aged 17-29 years, who were surveyed on dietary habits, smoking, physical activity, previous illnesses and nutritional status. Of which 47% did not have breakfast and 35% did not have lunch every day, they also consumed low amounts of vegetables (51.2%), fruits (39.4%) and milk products (57.5%), 66% were sedentary, 40.3% smoked and 27.4% were overweight; the frequency of consumption of soft drinks, chips, cakes and sweets were very high, and obesity was present. In conclusion, the food grant has some positive effects, despite socio-economic differences.

Becerra, Pinzón and Vargas7, in their cross-sectional study, in order to determine the nutritional status and some characteristics of food consumption of undergraduate students at the Faculty of Medicine of the National University of Colombia admitted during the 2010-II and 2011-I semesters, anthropometry was performed (weight, height and waist circumference) and an instrument was applied that included socioeconomic variables, frequency of consumption of certain foods and meal times. A total of 199 students were surveyed, 71.9% of whom were male and 28.1% female, with the result that malnutrition was slightly higher in males than in females, with a high frequency of soda, fast food and the addition of fat to food. In conclusion, the inadequate eating habits found in this study are directly related to the nutritional status of the population studied.

Campo et al8 developed the study entitled Healthy lifestyles and risk behaviours in medical students at the Institute of Higher Education in Bogotá (Colombia), where 651 medical students were evaluated in relation to their lifestyles, using the "Lifestyle questionnaire for young university students". The result was that, in this population, there are no healthy practices with respect to physical activity and leisure time. The conclusion is that healthy lifestyles are evident in most of the dimensions evaluated, suggesting the proposal of strategies to promote activities that strengthen leisure time and motivate physical activity.

Tamayo et al9 , in their descriptive cross-sectional study, which aimed to identify the lifestyles of 205 randomly selected university students from a Faculty of Dentistry in the city of Cali (Colombia), to whom the "Lifestyle Questionnaire" was applied.

Vida de Jóvenes Universitarios" (Life of Young University Students), which assessed eight dimensions of lifestyle. The results showed that the healthiest practice was physical activity (30.8%) and the most risky were interpersonal skills (73.5%), sleep (72.2%) and alcohol, cigarettes and illegal drugs (70.6%). In conclusion, physical activity was the healthiest practice in women than in men; however, women had higher risk practices such as alcohol, cigarette and illegal drugs consumption.

Atucha et al10 , in their cross-sectional descriptive study with the aim of analysing the lifestyles of students of the Degree in Pharmacy at the University of Murcia - Spain, evaluated students enrolled in the first, second, third, fourth and fifth years during the 2015/2016 academic year. The study concluded that the majority of students have a good quality of life, although habits such as smoking and alcohol consumption tend to worsen during university life.

At the national level, Barrenechea et al11 , in their cross-sectional exploratory study where they determined the degree of daytime sleepiness and sleep quality in 195 and 199 third and fourth year medical students respectively, at the "Universidad San Martin de Porres de Lima" (Peru) in 2010, using the Epworth Sleepiness Scale and the Modified Pittsburgh Sleep Quality Index, the overall result was that 80% and 47% of students had 6 or less hours and 5 or less hours of sleep respectively, which shows that there is a very poor quality of sleep with a high frequency and excessive sleepiness during the day in the study population.

Becerra12 , in his descriptive study where he evaluated the role of coping in the relationship between perceived stress and health behaviours of 155 first-year students at a private university in Lima (Peru) in 2015. Using measures of perceived stress. The results showed that the hierarchical multiple regression analyses for the coping variable best predicted health behaviours, by

On the other hand, emotion-focused coping constituted a style that favourably affects the habits of alcohol, tobacco and other drug consumption, sleep and rest, and self-care and medical care, while avoidant coping does so unfavourably. In conclusion, the results of the present investigation serve as an aid in the design of programmes for promotion and prevention with the aim of encouraging the adoption of health behaviours among university students.

Vílchez et al13 , in their cross-sectional study where they determined the relationship between anxiety, stress and depression considered mental health problems and sleep quality in 1,040 university students of Human Medicine from eight faculties in Peru from the first to the sixth year of studies. It was found that 693 students (77.69%) slept inadequately. Regarding mental health, 290 (32.51%) were found to suffer from depression, 472 (52.91%) from anxiety and 309 (34.64%) from stress. It was concluded that, among second and third year students, there was a high frequency of poor sleepers and that poor sleep quality was associated with anxiety, depression and stress.

2.2. THEORETICAL AND SCIENTIFIC BASES

Before addressing the healthy lifestyles of an individual it is necessary to know that when talking about health there is also the counterpart which is disease, to which many people pay attention only when they are faced with a treatment and not before when they can implement prevention and health promotion, the WHO14 in 1948, defined health as "the complete state of physical, mental and social well-being and not merely the absence of disease". Each individual must be in a state of complete well-being to be considered well, however, to achieve this it is necessary to take into account the lifestyles that are practised; it can be said that lifestyle is a set of habits and behaviours that constitute protective factors for health or risk factors for disease, taking into account the way of life and living conditions.

During the 1980s there were attempts to give a concept to lifestyle, but so far there is no exact definition. Moreover, the terminology that exists between lifestyle in general and healthy lifestyle is still used synonymously by different authors today, despite the efforts of the
O.M.S. to differentiate them15.

However, different lifestyles can be considered; we have the healthy lifestyle, which is broken down into two dimensions with behaviours such as not consuming cigarettes or alcohol, as well as consuming healthy food, and another where activities such as sport, frequent exercise, maintaining low body mass indexes are included; in turn, we have the free lifestyle, which is characterised by behaviours that affect the individual such as alcohol consumption, consuming unhealthy food, having a lack of interest in physical appearance and, ultimately, the socialised lifestyle, which refers to how each society is organised with regard to access to information, and the socialised lifestyle, which refers to how each society organises itself with regard to access to information.

culture and education, i.e. a relationship between individual responsibility and social policies [14].

From the aforementioned classification we find habits that favour the development of a healthy lifestyle such as: physical culture, traffic culture, personal care, healthy eating habits, cultural habits in leisure time, responsible sexual practices and vaccination habits. There are also habits that do not contribute to the development of a healthy lifestyle, such as: consumption of drugs, cigarettes and/or alcohol, environmental pollution and inadequate nutrition [14].

It is important to consider that the beginnings of studies on the subject originated in the area of prevention of diseases affecting the heart and cardiovascular system, so the variables in these studies were risk behaviours for this type of disease, such as: alcohol and cigarette consumption, dietary habits and physical exercise. In addition, the samples of these studies were mainly made up of adults affected or not by these cardiovascular problems [15].

Thus, due to the continuous increase in the concern for health education, both the O.M.S as well as public organisations dedicated to improving the well-being of the population of children and young people, led to an increase in the number of studies where children and adolescents were included as samples, as well as an increase in the number of variables studied that were part of lifestyles. For this reason, the following habits are now included: adequate nutrition, physical exercise, adequate sleep patterns, safe behaviour and accident prevention, non-abuse of harmful substances (alcohol, illegal drugs, tobacco); adherence to medical treatment; and finally, adequate management of emotions and stress [15].

In 2008, the WHO defined exercise and physical activity as "those bodily movements and activities that require more energy consumption than is produced in a state of rest or when performing a cognitive activity that promotes health". It is known that both exercise and physical activity reduce the risk of coronary heart disease and prevent chronic diseases as part of a good lifestyle. Psychologically, they act in a positive way, as they help to regulate certain emotions, reduce states of anxiety, tension and depression, thus increasing the feeling of well-being [15].

According to Varela et al16 , moderate physical activity (i.e., that performed two to three times a week for at least 20 to 30 minutes), which produces an energy expenditure greater than 10% of that produced by daily activities, could serve as protective factors in avoiding a sedentary lifestyle. Activities such as playing outdoors, housework, climbing stairs, walking, cycling as a means of transport, sport or exercise could serve as protective factors in avoiding a sedentary lifestyle, as well as bringing some benefits such as: increased neuronal plasticity, elevation in the level of brain-derived neurotrophic factor, favouring visual memory and learning, activation of the sympathetic nervous system releasing noradrenaline and dopamine, which help to improve mood. It also positively influences school performance, especially in the area of mathematics and reading.

Physical activity can be vigorous, when the individual presents a significant increase in breathing or heart rate, with heavy sweating, lasting at least 20 minutes over a period of three days a week, and light physical activity, which is performed in free time, achieves sweating in the individual with a slight increase in breathing or heart rate, lasting at least 30 minutes and with a frequency of five days a week [17].

When addressing the dimension of eating habits, aspects linked to food intake and choice are considered, as well as: the type, quantity, times, places of consumption and practices to control weight. These actions satisfy the body's physical needs, favouring the functioning of its vital processes during the day, preventing the onset of certain diseases and thus improving the state of health15.

Inappropriate eating habits, stereotypes emphasising physical beauty and sexual debauchery have damaged eating behaviours in youth, contributing to eating disorders such as metabolic endocrinopathies, which then lead to heart disease (arrhythmias) and even death [15].

For this reason, proper nutrition is characterised by a balanced diet with all essential nutrients such as minerals, carbohydrates, vitamins and proteins. Recommended eating habits in this regard would be to reduce the consumption of fats, increase the intake of milk, vegetables, fruits and high-fibre foods and reduce the consumption of sugar, sweets and flour14.

In addition, it is recommended to reduce the consumption of animal-derived fats, increase the consumption of dairy products, tubers and especially vegetables, fruit and foods rich in fibre, reduce the intake of sugar, refined flours, sweets and do not consume alcoholic beverages in excess. Thus, a balanced diet should provide the basic nutrients and fibre necessary to meet needs, including foods from the four basic groups: fruit, cereals, vegetables, dairy products, meat and fish [18].

Eating habits are broad in nature and there are many cultural, economic and social factors that favour the maintenance and establishment of changes in food consumption behaviour. For this reason, these habits are contingent on the availability of food, economic resources and choice. Associated factors can be found within these three main areas. Food availability is influenced by the economic patterns of each country, geographical and climatic factors, transport and communication infrastructure, agricultural sector policies and, in a broader sense, food, nutrition and health policies [19].

The behaviours of each human being are conditioned by the environment, favouring them or making them easier or more difficult to practice, but still being able to influence this environment. From an integrative perspective, multiple conditioning factors are summarised on four levels: the individual (intrapersonal) level, where personal characteristics come into play; the psychological level (knowledge, attitudes, personal security, etc.); the biological level, where food preferences, taste sensitivity and education of the sense of taste are included; the behavioural level, where a habitual eating pattern is worked on, personal perceptions such as adaptation to a personal situation, organisation of daily life, among others19 .

The social environment (interpersonal) where there is the family, the school, the group of friends and their respective interactions; the physical environment (community) where the accessibility and availability of food, school canteen, fast-food, sweet shop, food, vending machines, among others are considered; the macrosystem (society), where advertising, marketing, social and cultural norms, food production and distribution systems, policies and regulations related to food, prices, distribution, availability, among others, are framed [19].

For the normality of a diet to be judged, it would take several generations. For this reason and for practical purposes, rules have been created which a priori make it possible to know the normality of a diet. These rules are called The first, called the law of quantity, explains that the quantity of food must cover the calorie requirements of the organism and maintain the balance of its equilibrium; in the second, the law of quality, it is mentioned that the diet must be complete in its composition in order to offer the organism, which is an indivisible unit, all the substances that make it up; thirdly, the law of harmony, which refers to the relationship between the quantities of the various nutritional principles that make up the diet, and lastly, the law of adequacy, which states that the purpose of the diet is subject to its suitability for the organism [19].

It is important to consider that the nutritional requirement "is the smallest amount of a nutrient that must be absorbed or consumed on average by an individual over a given period of time (depending on each nutrient) to maintain adequate nutrition". The determination of their nutritional recommendations is established by assessing the average basal requirement of a nutrient absorbed. Both requirements and recommendations vary according to body weight, height, age and sex of the individual and are calculated on the basis of moderate physical activity [19].

Dietary fibre has been defined as "the sum of polysaccharides and lignin present in vegetables that cannot be digested by the endogenous secretions of the gastrointestinal tract". Regarding fibre intake in a diet, it is estimated that it should be 25-35 grams per day or 10-13 grams/1 000 kilocalories. This amount is achieved by consuming fruits, vegetables, legumes and whole grains, with an insoluble/soluble ratio of 3/1 usually [19].

Carina19 states that calcium must be included as another element of an adequate diet. Calcium is found in the body in an amount ranging from 1,100 to 1,200 grams, 99% of which is found in the bones, while the remaining 1% is stored in the plasma. Physiologically about 45% is bound mainly to albumin, while 47% is found as ionised or free calcium and the remaining material creates citrate and calcium phosphate complexes. He also states that "Adequate calcium intake according to the National Academy of Sciences (N.A.S.) of the United States (U.S.) should be 1000 mg/day for adult men and women".

In this context, nutrition is a voluntary and educable process. A constant in the life of a human being and his or her social environment is given by the food-nutrition binomial, which is why an adequate diet ensures an optimal nutritional state and therefore generates a healthy eating habit [19].

It has been recommended that with regard to the type of food, the consumption of fruit and vegetables per day should be five portions; considering once a day, the consumption of raw vegetables and fresh fruit; also consume white and red meats (chicken and fish) leaving aside visible fat three to four times a week. Also, increase the intake of fish, whether sea or river, and stop eating cold meats and sausages. It is important to reduce the intake of sugar and salt, and to avoid sodas, alcoholic beverages and artificial sweets. For this reason, it is always preferable to consume water (at least 2 litres during the day, always using drinking water) and natural juices. Another recommendation is to increase the intake of a variety of pasta, pulses and cereals, and to consume cakes, biscuits, biscuits and other products in moderation. It should also be emphasised that drinking water should be used for washing and preparing food. Finally, it should be mentioned that sufficient amounts of each type of food are needed on a daily basis. For this reason, a well-served breakfast and eating throughout the day, at various times of the day, is a good idea.

servings (4 servings being recommended), in order to improve digestion without losing vital energy [19].

Sleep is an active, rhythmic physiological state that alternates with the other basic state of wakefulness, which occurs every 24 hours. Its optimal duration is on average 7 to 8 h in a young person, and its loss is considered an important social problem in modern times, especially for medical students, as a result of the academic load at university. It should be noted that sleep promotes bodily recovery and facilitates the learning and memory process. For this reason, the quality of sleep should be assessed from two aspects: quantitative (number of awakenings during the night, sleep latency and sleep duration) and qualitative (feeling rested upon awakening, sleep depth and overall satisfaction with sleep) [20].

Studies affirm that both the quality and quantity of sleep is associated with academic performance. Despite this, it is customary to reduce sleep time, which generates states of stress, anxiety and depression, affecting academic activities during the day. The university training stage conditions the generation of stress, a situation that overloads students due to the long academic hours; for this reason, encouraging the use of psychosocial coping resources is insufficient, as in the long term it conditions the appearance of somatic and mental disorders or social maladjustment [20].

At university, due to overloaded timetables, teachers and their academic demands and competitiveness among classmates, anxiety is the psychological disorder par excellence, which is preceded by fear and stress. Similarly, the most recurrent psychological syndrome in this case is depression, which is represented by low mood accompanied by appetite and sleep disorders [20].

Problems resulting from poor sleep affect both physically and psychologically, and studies have shown that such chronic sleep problems are related to an increased risk of depression and anxiety, which are considered to be insomnia-producing disorders [20]. It is a broad term, extremely current and interesting, which currently still does not have a consensus definition [21].

According to the Canadian physiologist Selye, quoted by Cano22 , the definition of the term stress has been very controversial from the moment that interest in its study began. It is understood as "an individual's reaction or response to physiological changes, emotional or behavioural reactions, as well as a stimulus (capable of provoking a stress reaction), as well as the interaction between the characteristics of the stimulus and the individual's resources".

This approach is currently accepted as the most accurate. It considers stress as a consequence of an imbalance between the demands of the environment (internal or external stressors) and the resources of the individual. Thus, the elements that interact with stressful situations are both situational (e.g. in the workplace) and individual variables of the subject facing the situation and its consequences [22].

In this complex phenomenon, interrelated variables are considered: academic stressors, subjective experience of stress, moderators of academic stress and finally, effects of academic stress. All of these appear in the same organisational environment: the university. In particular, the university represents a set of highly stressful situations because the individual may experience, even temporarily, a lack of control over the new environment, potentially

stressor, in combination with other factors, can lead to academic failure [21].

The scarce amount of work on the subject shows that there are notable rates of stress in the university population, which reaches higher levels in the early years of the degree course and in the stages prior to exams. Contributing factors include biological factors such as age and gender, psychosocial factors (social support, coping strategies, Type A behaviour pattern), psycho-socio-educational factors (academic self-concept, courses, type of studies) and socio-economic factors (enjoyment of scholarships, place of residence). These variables influence the process of stress, from the appearance of the factors that cause it until its consequences are expressed, so that one or the other may favour a better coping with the stressor [21].

Stress as a process can have short and long term consequences, academically it affects the emotional, physical and interpersonal relationships, and is experienced differently by each individual. After reviewing research on academic stress, it is possible to distinguish three main levels where its effects are felt: behavioural, cognitive and physiological. These include short- and long-term effects [21].

On the behavioural level, lifestyle changes as the assessment period approaches, leading to unhealthy habits (excessive consumption of caffeine, hallucinogenic substances, tobacco, even the ingestion of tranquillisers), which will then lead to mental health disorders [21].

On a cognitive level, emotions and appraisal of reality are substantially modified before taking exams and afterwards when grades are announced. Also, the subjective perception of stress increases during the exam period, which is more important than the time of the exams.

outside of it. Finally, at the psychophysiological level, suppression of T-cell and *natural killer cell* (NKC) activity during exam periods (situations perceived as highly stressful) has been documented in students. These changes indicate immune suppression and thus increased vulnerability to illness on the part of the body. It has been confirmed that there are immune changes related to academic stress, with poor T-lymphocyte response to mitogens [21].

The consumption of toxic substances (illegal drugs, alcohol and tobacco) refers to the consumption, application or assimilation of these substances, which generate variations at the level of the central nervous centre, modifying behaviour. Such changes are related to immediate effects when consumed, producing negative health consequences at the cardiovascular and colon level, academic and/or work-related problems, unwanted pregnancies, road accidents, infectious and contagious diseases, suicide, violence and mental health problems15.

In universities there is a risk of drug and alcohol consumption by university students, as there are factors that influence the consumption of these substances such as: Low self-esteem, academic stress, easy access to these substances, lack of preventive or student support programmes, organisational culture that accepts and facilitates consumption [14].

It should be noted that cigarette smoking is an increasing phenomenon in adolescents and young adults. It predisposes to premature acute myocardial infarction (AMI), probably due to the stimulus of spasm in healthy coronary arteries. Likewise, frequent consumption is recorded in young patients with coronary heart disease, 96% of whom had been consumers until the event appeared, and there is also a relationship with advanced coronary atherosclerosis in this same type of population [18].

On the other hand, passive smokers such as children present respiratory symptoms and adults death from lung cancer. Young people can produce endothelial malfunction in large calibre arteries depending on the dose, similar to the degree of vascular impairment also found in active smokers of the same age group. A relationship with pathophysiological expressions has been seen with even short term exposure to tobacco smoke. In addition, the lipid profile may be toxically altered and may be associated with a decrease in the intima-media *thickness* (IMT) of the common carotid artery [18].

It is known that alcohol intake increases during adolescence and young adulthood, particularly during periods outside school, and decreases as people approach their thirties. The effects on health depend on the amount of alcohol consumed and patterns of consumption, typically the J-curve, which shows the damage that alcohol causes to health. The J-curve describes that a decrease in alcohol consumption is associated with a reduction in overall mortality by up to 18% and in heart and vascular disease by 30%. In addition, heavy drinking is associated with a risk of cerebrovascular disease (CVD), and in direct association with smoking increases the overall mortality rate [18].

On the other hand, a phenomenon that has acquired great relevance is the consumption of drugs (heroin, cocaine, marijuana, among others) considered illegal and legal (alcohol, tobacco and prescription drugs). These generate health problems, including different types of cancers, respiratory diseases, heart disease and CVD. According to drug dependence, one of the many existing classifications differentiates between legal and illegal drugs18 .

For Fernanda and Oviedo18 legal substances are those whose sale and consumption are permitted by law. Examples par excellence of these are tobacco and alcohol, which are categorised as institutionalised drugs, as well as being the most widely consumed and generating social and health problems. Undoubtedly, the main cause of preventable death in the world is tobacco consumption, causing a total of three million deaths per year. More than all those caused by alcohol, illegal drugs, homicides, suicides, car accidents and Acquired Immune Deficiency Syndrome (A.I.D.S.) combined. For this reason, the sale and use of illegal drugs has no legal recommendation.

In the last decade, these drugs have created too many serious problems in different societies. These problems are mainly of a social nature, not related to physical health. People who die from illegal drugs and their effects are very few compared to those from alcohol and tobacco. Both legal and illegal drugs are a relevant health hazard18 .

However, illegal drugs present both pharmacological effects and certain risks, unlike legal drugs. For example, they can be sold under the label of a drug that is in fact a very different drug; with such diverse compounds that they can in themselves be more harmful to the integrity of the person; in addition to the existence of insufficient health measures when they are administered; those who consume them are often unsure of the dose, whether for reasons of economy, demand or other situations. This also brings with it social conflicts, as drug users generate drug trafficking, public insecurity, assaults, robberies and so on. In addition to generating employment and economic problems18.

2.3. DEFINITION OF BASIC TERMINOLOGIES

1. Lifestyle. - These are the habitual, everyday behaviours that characterise an individual's way of life and are usually permanent over time" [23].

2. Physical activity. - Physical activity is defined as any activity involving bodily movement produced by skeletal muscles and which produces significant energy expenditure.

3. Eating habits. - These are habits that are learned throughout life, i.e. they are maintained, but may change according to lifestyle" [24].

4. Sleep. - It is a necessary and restorative physiological state, usually periodic and reversible, characterised by a depression of the senses, of consciousness, of spontaneous motility, in which the person can be awakened by sensory stimuli" [24].

5. Stress. - Process that is initiated by a set of environmental demands that the individual receives, to which he/she must give an adequate response, using his/her coping resources" [22].

6. Harmful substances. - A generic name that has been found in the literature to refer to the use of alcohol, tobacco, inhalants, other drugs and pharmaceuticals" [25].

CHAPTER III

MATERIAL AND METHODS

3.1. Place of execution

It was held at the Professional School of Obstetrics of the National University of Tumbes.

3.2. Type and design of research

a) Type of research:

The research work is of a simple descriptive and cross-sectional type.

b) Research design:

The research corresponds to a non-experimental design, with a quantitative, cross-sectional, descriptive methodological approach, the research design is descriptive - non-experimental, corresponding to the following scheme:

The simple scheme is as follows:

$$M \longrightarrow OXi$$

Where:

M: Students enrolled in the academic semester 2018 - I. O: Observation of the variable.

Xi: Lifestyle.

3.3. Population, sample and sampling

a. Population: The population consisted of the total number of students enrolled up to the academic semester 2018 - I, making a total of 230 students.

b. Sample population:

We worked with the effective sample population considered at the time of applying the instrument and then applying the inclusion and exclusion criteria (128 students):

Table of students enrolled up to the academic year 2018 - I			
Students	Cycle	Meet Inclusion criteria	Does not meet inclusion criteria
Regular	I		-
	II	Not applicable	
	III		-
	IV		-
	V	29	1
	VI	1	1
	VII		
	VIII		
Interns	IX	-	
	X	-	
Laggards		-	63
Total			102

Total number of students surveyed who underwent data processing.

c) Unit of analysis: The unit of analysis will be made up of each of the students of the School of Obstetrics of the National University of Tumbes who met the selection criteria for the sample.

3.4. Inclusion and exclusion criteria

Inclusion:

- We considered the 2014 - I to 2018 - I intake years of the School of Midwifery who, after informed consent, voluntarily agreed to participate in the study.

Exclusion:

- Students from the entry years 2000 - I to 2013 - II.
- Students in the IX and X cycles because they are doing their academic internship.
- Students who were not present or arrived after the start of the questionnaire application.
- Those who find it difficult to answer the questionnaire   the questionnaire.
- Those who were indisposed did not wish to participate in the survey.

3.5. Methods, techniques and instruments of data collection Method: The

survey was used to explore objectively and at the same time to obtain information from a number of different sources.
considerable number of people during the course of the research. The surveys allow data to be standardised for further analysis, at low cost and in a short period of time.

Technique: It was the interview, which is a situation of interrelation or dialogue between people, in this case between the interviewer and the interviewee.

Instrument: It was a questionnaire created by Bennasar M. [4], called "Lifestyle questionnaire for young university students version 2 (CEVJU - R2)" which was modified according to the reality of the Tumbes region. This questionnaire is anonymous and consists of two parts: general data and research data.

The first section is the general data of the students themselves, such as year of entry, current academic semester, sex and age. In the second section called research data, 4 dimensions were evaluated (physical activity, eating habits, sleep - stress and consumption of toxic substances), adapted from the CEVJU-R2, consisting of 26 questions, of which 3 are from the dimension of physical activity, 10 from eating habits, 5 referring to sleep and stress, and 8 with respect to the consumption of toxic substances, which were elaborated based on the variables that proved to be more influential in the lifestyle, also because of the objectives of the research.

Likewise, to award the score to each question, it was considered that only when the measurement scale was nominal, the maximum and minimum score (2 and 0 points respectively) was awarded to the answer to the questions (question 6, question 7, question 16, question 19, question 21, question 23, question 24, question 25 and question 26); for the other answers to the questions with ordinal measurement scale (question 1, question 2, question 3, question 4, question 5, question 8, question 9, question 10, question 11, question 12, question 13, question 14, question 15, question 17, question 18, question 20, question 22) the maximum, intermediate and minimum score was given (2,1 and 0 respectively). For more details see table N° 01 of annex N° 05.

Validity and reliability: The modified instrument used was validated by expert judgement, by a health professional, who, using a validation sheet (Annex 03), evaluated and provided recommendations. The resulting version was subjected to a pilot test with 10 students from the School of Nursing, as they had similar characteristics to the target population. To measure the internal consistency or reliability of the instrument, Cronbach's Alpha Coefficient was used, which had an acceptable value of 0.84, which supports the instrument applied. (Annex N° 04).

3.6. Data processing and analysis plan

Data collection procedure:

After approval of the project, permission was requested from the authorities of the School of Obstetrics of the Faculty of Health Sciences - National University of Tumbes.

The anonymous lifestyle questionnaire was administered on the premises of the School of Midwifery to students with informed consent.

For the collection of data, the classrooms were visited during the corresponding timetables of the subjects of the speciality, ensuring the participation of regularly enrolled students, the respective authorisation for the execution of the project was presented to the teachers who taught their classes and, once the pass was given, the objectives of the research were explained in detail; then the student was given the informed consent form and the research questionnaire, which was seen and read by the student himself, who signed it, agreeing to participate and to develop it. We proceeded to apply the instrument to the total number of students in the class, in the planned time of 15 minutes including the reading and signing of the informed consent, the environment where it was applied was quiet and free of interference for an adequate resolution of the same; then each of the questionnaires were kept in a sealed envelope for their respective processing according to the sample and selected criteria.

Data processing and analysis:

Once the data had been collected, each of the instruments was coded and each one was checked to ensure that it was correctly filled in, separating those that had errors that made it impossible to interpret correctly according to inclusion and exclusion criteria.

For the interpretation of the lifestyles according to the data collected, the SPSS programme was used with the scale method, by means of which a maximum score of 45 and a minimum of 20 with a mean of 31 was assigned, which was used to elaborate the score ranges, which were used to qualify whether a lifestyle was healthy or unhealthy.

For the interpretation of each dimension, a score was assigned based on the number and type of questions assigned to it (see table No. 01 in annex No. 05), contemplated in the assessment scale of the table of operationalisation of variables, where the sum of the points per dimension is interpreted as follows:

LIFESTYLE DIMENSION RATING SCALE

Dimension	Indicators (scores)	
Physical Activity	0 - 3 pts. (inadequate)	4 - 6 pts. (appropriate)
Eating Habits	0 - 10 pts. (inadequate)	11 - 20 pts. (appropriate)
Sleep-Stress	0 - 5 pts. (inadequate)	6 - 10 pts. (optimal)
Toxic Substance Use	0 - 8 pts. (consumer)	9 - 16 pts. (non-consumer)

3.6. Ethical Aspects

This research was carried out in an ethical environment considering the 3 fundamental principles that are included in most ethical codes and norms: the principle of beneficence, respect for human dignity and the principle of justice [26].

Principle of non-maleficence

This includes no harm, it is not acceptable to expose research participants to experiences that are seriously or permanently harmful; in the present study, students from the School of Midwifery were not exposed to psychological harm. Throughout the course of the research, they were protected from any situation that would make them uncomfortable answering the questions. The information was not used for purposes other than those stated26.

Principle of respect for human dignity

It refers to the right of midwifery students to decide to participate voluntarily in the study without risk of reprisal or detrimental treatment; it also means that they can terminate their participation at any time, refuse to provide information, and not be coerced in any way. In this research the students decided to participate in the research on a voluntary basis26.

Principle of justice

It encompasses the right of students to fair and equitable treatment before, during and after their participation, including aspects such as: fair and non-discriminatory selection of subjects, so that both risks and benefits are shared equitably, non-judgmental treatment of those who refused to participate, respectful and kind treatment at all times, and consideration of the honourable nature of the agreements made between researcher and researched26.

CHAPTER IV

RESULTS

Table N° 1

PHYSICAL ACTIVITY CARRIED OUT BY STUDENTS OF THE SCHOOL OF OBSTETRICS OF THE NATIONAL UNIVERSITY OF TUMBES - 2018

Physical Activity	N
Adequate	69.5
Sedentary	30.5
Total	100

Source: Author's survey of students at the School of Midwifery.

Regarding physical activity, 69.5% of the students surveyed were physically active, while 30.5% were sedentary.

Table N° 1 - A

TYPE, FREQUENCY AND TIME OF PHYSICAL EXERCISE PERFORMED BY STUDENTS OF THE SCHOOL OF OBSTETRICS OF THE NATIONAL UNIVERSITY OF TUMBES - 2018

Type of physical exercise performed		N
Does not engage in any activity		30.5
They practice some kind of activity:		69.5
-Just one exercise	18/14.1%	
Walking minimum 30 min25/19. 5% - Walking minimum 30 min25/19. 5% - Walking minimum 30 min25/19. 5% - Walking minimum 30 min		
-Aerobics	07/5.5%	
-Futbol	06/4.7%	
Volleyball	07/5.5%	
Cycling	13/10.2%	
Lifting weights	06/4.7%	
-Swimming	07/5.5%	

Frequency of physical exercise		N
Non-practising		30.5
Other times per week and every day		69.5
1-2 times per week	38/30%	
3-4 times a week	26/20%	
5-6 times per week	13/10%	
Every day		

Time allocated for physical exercise		N
Non-practising		30.5
Other amount of time		69.5
-15-30 min	51/40%	
30-45 min/ more than 45 min 38/29.5% -30-45 min/ more than 45 min 38/29.5% -30-45 min/ more than 45 min		

TOTAL	100

Source: Author's survey of students at the School of Midwifery.

Table N° 2

EATING HABITS OF THE STUDENTS OF THE SCHOOL OF OBSTETRICS
OF THE NATIONAL UNIVERSITY OF TUMBES - 2018

Eating Habits	N	
Adequate	77	
Inadequate	51	
Total		100

Source: Author's survey of students at the School of Midwifery.

With regard to eating habits, of the total number of students surveyed, 60% were adequate and 40% were inadequate.

Table N° 2 - A

TYPE, FREQUENCY AND QUANTITY OF FOOD CONSUMPTION OF STUDENTS OF THE SCHOOL OF OBSTETRICS OF THE NATIONAL UNIVERSITY OF TUMBES - 2018

Fast food consumption		N	
Always			30
in some cases			30
Never		51	
Times per day of fibre intake		N	
Does not consume		51	
Consume other times a day		77	
1-2 times a day	21/16%		
3-4 times a day	20/16%		
5-6 times a day	18/14%		
-more than 6 times	18/14%		
Fruit consumption in a typical week		N	
does not eat fruit		51	
does eat fruit		77	
Frequency of fruit consumption		N	
does not consume		51	
1-2 times per week	13/10%		
3-4 times a week	06/5%		
5-6 times per week	06/5%		
-every day	52/40%		
Units of fruit consumed in a day normal		N	
does not consume		51	
Consume another number of units in a day		77	
1-3 units per day	33/25%		
3-5 units per day	12/10%		
5-7 units per day	06/5%		
more than 7 units per day 26/20% -more than 7 units per day 26/20% -more than 7 units per day 26/20% -more than 7 units per day 26/20			
TOTAL			100

Source: Author's survey of students at the School of Midwifery.

Table N° 2 - B

TYPE, FREQUENCY AND QUANTITY OF FOOD CONSUMPTION OF STUDENTS OF THE SCHOOL OF OBSTETRICS OF THE NATIONAL UNIVERSITY OF TUMBES - 2018

		N
Frequency of soda consumption		N
Times per week that you consume soft drinks		51
2 times a week	25/20%	
3-5 times per week13/10% -3-5 times per week13/10% -3-5 times per week		
6 times a week	13/10	
Never		77
Days on which you consumed soda in the previous week		N
Number of days (1 to more than 6)		51
-More than 6 days	00/00%	
-3-5 days	20/16%	
-1-2 days	31/24%	
Does not consume		77
Number of bottles of soft drinks consumed per day		N
Number of bottles consumed per day		51
5-6 bottles per day	00/00%	
3-5 bottles per day	00/00%	
1-2 bottles per day	51/40%	
None		77
Daily water intake (no juices, soft drinks, soups)		N
If you drink water		77
Does not drink water		51
Number of glasses of water consumed per day		N
Does not consume		51
Number of glasses consumed per day		77
- < of 4 glasses	19/15%	
- 6-8 glasses	19/15%	
- > of 8 glasses	39/30%	
TOTAL		100

Source: Author's survey of students at the School of Midwifery.

Table N° 3

SLEEP - STRESS IN THE STUDENTS OF THE SCHOOL OF OBSTETRICS OF
THE NATIONAL UNIVERSITY OF TUMBES - 2018

Sleep - Stress	N
Optimum	30
Inadequate	70
Total	100

Source: Author's survey of students at the School of Midwifery.

Regarding sleep - stress, 30% of the total number of students surveyed were optimal, while 70% were inadequate.

APPEARANCE, FREQUENCY OF SLEEP AND CAUSE OF STRESS IN STUDENTS OF THE SCHOOL OF OBSTETRICS OF THE NATIONAL UNIVERSITY OF TUMBES - 2018

Number of hours of sleep in a typical day	N	
< 6 hours		45
7-8 hours		30
> 8 hours		25
Number of hours of sleep in a day of university	N	
< 6 hours		45
7-8 hours		30
> than 8 hours		25
Presence of stress symptoms	N	
if you show symptoms of stress		70
no symptoms of stress		30
Stress by type of situation	N	
Type of stressful situation		70
partial reviews15/12% - partial reviews15/12% - partial reviews15/12% - partial reviews15/12% - partial reviews15/12% - partial reviews Academic overload40/31% - Overloaded40/31% -Overloaded40/31% - Overloaded40/31% -Overloaded Family problems12/9% -Family problems12/9% -Family problems12/9% - Family problems12/9% -Family problems -problems with my partner05/4% -problems with my partner05/4% -problems with my partner economic problems17/13% -economic problems		
None		30
Frequency of stress caused by previous situation	N	
always/almost always/often		
rarely		
Never		30
TOTAL		100

Source: Author's survey of students at the School of Midwifery.

Table N° 4

CONSUMPTION OF TOXIC SUBSTANCES IN STUDENTS OF THE
SCHOOL OF OBSTETRICS OF THE NATIONAL UNIVERSITY OF
TUMBES - 2018

Substance use toxins	N	
Non-consumers	25	
Consumers	103	80
Total		100

Source: Author's survey of students at the School of Midwifery.

With regard to substance use, of the total number of students surveyed, 20% are
non-users while 80% are users.

Table N° 4 - A

TYPE, FREQUENCY AND AMOUNT OF CONSUMPTION OF TOXIC SUBSTANCES IN STUDENTS OF THE SCHOOL OF OBSTETRICS OF THE NATIONAL UNIVERSITY OF TUMBES - 2018

Smoking habit	N	
Yes, it consumes	103	80
Does not consume	25	
Number of cigarettes consumed per day	N	
5-10 cigarettes/more than 10 cigarettes	58	45
less than 5	45	35
No response	25	
Consumes alcoholic beverages	N	
does consume	103	80
does not consume	25	
Frequency of drinking alcoholic beverages	N	
3-4 times per week/ 5 or more times per week	45	35
1-2 times per week	58	45
rarely	25	
He was suggested to take some kind of drug.	N	
if you were proposed	103	80
you were not proposed	25	
Knows people who use drugs of some kind	N	
does know	103	80
does not know	25	
Used drugs of any kind	N	
did occasionally use	103	80
did not use occasionally	25	
Do you currently use any type of drug	N	
does currently consume	103	80
does not currently consume	25	
TOTAL		100

Source: Author's survey of students at the School of Midwifery.

LIFESTYLE ACCORDING TO ITS DIMENSIONS OF THE
STUDENTS OF THE SCHOOL OF OBSTETRICS OF THE
NATIONAL UNIVERSITY OF TUMBES - 2018

	Physical Activity	Eating Habits	Sleep - Stress	Substance use Toxins		X%
	n	N	n	N		X%
HEALTHY	70	51	30	25		44.875
UNHEALTHY	31	77	70	103	80	55.125
TOTAL	100	100	100	100		100

Source: Author's survey of students at the School of Midwifery.

Healthy lifestyles in the students of the School of Obstetrics predominate in the dimensions of physical activity and eating habits with 70% and 60%; likewise, unhealthy lifestyles prevail in the dimensions of sleep-stress and consumption of toxic substances with 70% and 80%. Meanwhile, unhealthy lifestyles prevail on average with 55.125%.

CHAPTER V

DISCUSSION

When addressing the physical activity dimension, exercise and physical activity are considered to be those body movements and activities that require a higher energy consumption than that produced in a state of rest or when carrying out a cognitive activity that favours health, psychologically they act in a positive way, as they help to regulate certain emotions, reduce states of anxiety, tension and depression, thus increasing the feeling of wellbeing [15.]

It is also explained that regular physical exercise, carried out in an appropriate manner, helps to maintain a stable weight, as well as improving the state of the body and mind; helping us to maintain cardiovascular, musculoskeletal and metabolic function27. Thus, in the present study, 69.5% of the respondents in relation to physical activity practised, while 30.5% did not (Table 02). Similar data were found in the study by Bennasar M., carried out at the University of the Balearic Islands in Spain, entitled Lifestyles in University Students, which concluded that 65.8% of university students stated that they did physical activity4.

Likewise, one of the weaknesses found in the lifestyles of these populations is the practice of exercise; despite being aware of its relevance in preventing cardiovascular diseases and its general benefits for physical and mental health2. In the same vein, it was found that of the population studied who do some type of physical activity, 30% reported doing physical activity 1 to 2 times a week, 20% 3 to 4 times a week, while 10% 5 to 6 times a week and every day (Table No. 02 - A). Contrary to what was described in the study by Atucha N. et al, at the University of Murcia, entitled Health styles and healthy habits in students of the Degree in Pharmacy, it was concluded that 61.9% of them claim to do physical activity between 2 and 6 times a week and every day (Table N° 02 - A).

3 times a week, 19.8% only once a week and 13.5% of students claim to do physical exercise more than 4 times a week10 .

Nowadays, the lack of physical activity is compounded by other harmful habits of the contemporary lifestyle (overeating, smoking, stress, inadequate use of leisure time, drug addiction, among others), which unleashes a second epidemiological revolution, where chronic degenerative diseases predominate over acute infectious diseases. Physical activity has the potential to reduce risk factors for chronic diseases and to generate positive changes with respect to other risk factors for these diseases2.

It can be said that most of the students interviewed do physical activity, giving the impression that they exercise, but the problem lies in the fact that they do not do it with the correct frequency and time, which means that the physical exercise is not adequate. This is reflected in the physical activity dimension table, where 30.5% still do not practice physical activity (Table N° 02).

With regard to the eating habits dimension, this considers aspects linked to the selection, ingestion, type and quantity of food, the times and places in which it is consumed and some practices associated with weight control16 . Eating habits are complex in nature and there are many social, cultural and economic factors that favour the establishment, maintenance and changes in food consumption patterns [19].

The data reveal that, with respect to the eating habits of the total number of students at the School of Midwifery, 60% are adequate, while 40% are inadequate (Table N° 03). These results are not similar to the study carried out by Ratner G., in 54 higher education centres throughout Chile, entitled Quality of nutrition and nutritional status in university students in 11 regions of Chile, where they concluded that there was a high prevalence of of inadequate eating and physical activity patterns in these well-educated young people6.

It was also found that students consume fruit (60%), but always eat fast food, pizza, fried chicken, hamburgers (30%) (Table N° 02 - A), they also consume 1 - 2 bottles of soft drinks a day (40%), twice a week (20%) (Table N° 02 - B). These results differ from the study carried out by Becerra12 , at the National University of Colombia called nutritional status and food consumption of university students admitted to the career of Medicine, where they conclude that the inadequate eating habits found are related to the nutritional status of the students. The prevalence of malnutrition is evidenced by the high frequency of consumption of fast food (29.1%), soft drinks 2 to 3 times a week (26.7%), daily fried food (12.5%) and the addition of fat to food (27.7%).

This reality is increasing every day in the considerable number of students who consume food with a high content of saturated fats and sugars, thus increasing the number of overweight people, a problem that currently contributes to the appearance of metabolic diseases such as obesity, which will lead in the future to more cases of diabetics in our environment. Although a large percentage of students at the School of Midwifery maintain an adequate consumption of fruit, this does not guarantee that this percentage will be maintained in the long term. 40% of students were found to have inadequate eating habits, with a clear risk possibly due to the pace of life involved in university work (table No. 03).

Regarding the dimension of sleep and stress, studies indicate that both the quality and quantity of sleep are related to academic performance. Knowingly, it is customary to sleep for less time than normal, which generates processes of anxiety, stress and depression, affecting academic activities during the day. For this reason, the university education stage is considered to be a determining factor for the generation of stress, a situation that can overburden students due to excessive academic hours, which, despite the use of psychosocial coping resources, can lead to mental and somatic disorders and even social maladjustment20 .

On analysing the instrument in the sleep quality - stress item, it was found that 30% were optimal, while 70% were inadequate (Table N° 03), on comparing these results with those of the study carried out by Barrenechea L. et al, at the University of San Martín de Porres, on sleep quality and excessive daytime sleepiness in third and fourth year medical students, similarities can be seen with the overall result of 80% and 47% of students with 6 or fewer hours and 5 or fewer hours respectively, indicating a high frequency of poor sleep quality and excessive daytime sleepiness in the medical students surveyed (unhealthy lifestyle)[11.]

When analysing the hours of sleep, it was found that the students to whom the questionnaire was applied answered that most of them slept < 6 hours in a normal day (45%) and 7 - 8 hours in a university day (30%) (Table N° 03 - A). These data were compared with the study carried out by Trujillo and Wilman at the Universidad del Atlántico in Medellín, entitled "Sleep and time allocation among students at the Universidad del Atlántico", which concluded that the optimal choice of sleep for students at this university is between 5.57 and 12 hours a day5. Also in relation to stress, they reported having symptoms of stress (70%) (Table N° 03 - A). When this result was compared, it was found to differ from that of the study carried out by Vílchez et al. on medical students at eight Peruvian universities, entitled Mental health and sleep quality in students at eight human medicine faculties in Peru, which concluded that, of the entire student population evaluated, they suffered from depression (32.51%), anxiety (52.91%) and stress (34.64%)[13.]

There is no doubt that within the population studied there is a tendency to academic stress which predisposes them in the future to a number of different health problems, because it affects emotional, physical and interpersonal relationships, which are experienced in different ways by people.

When addressing the dimension of toxic substances, it is worth mentioning that their consumption (alcohol, tobacco and illegal drugs) refers to the ingestion, application and absorption of these substances, which degenerate the central nervous centre and behaviour15. Furthermore, in universities, there is a risk of university students consuming alcoholic beverages and psychoactive substances, as there are factors that influence the consumption of these substances, such as: Low self-esteem, academic stress, easy access to these substances, lack of preventive or student support programmes and organisational culture that accepts and facilitates consumption16.

Of the total number of obstetric students, 20% are not consumers and 80% are consumers of toxic substances (Table N° 04), these data are similar to those of the study carried out by Campo et al, in a Higher Education Institution in Bogota called "healthy lifestyles and risk behaviours in medical students"; who concluded that those interviewed were at low risk (35%), moderate risk (84%), and high or severe risk (16%), with risky practices (unhealthy lifestyles) such as the consumption of alcohol, tobacco and illegal psychoactive substances (70.6%)[8].

A more detailed analysis of this dimension found students who claimed to be smokers (80%), to consume alcoholic beverages (80%) and to have occasionally consumed some type of drug (80%) (Table 4 - A). These results are similar in some respects to those of the study carried out by Atucha et al. at the University of Murcia entitled "health styles and healthy habits in students of the Degree in Pharmacy", who concluded that students have a mostly good quality of life, although habits such as smoking (25%) and alcohol consumption (93%) are evident and have a clear tendency to worsen during university life10 .

From the above, it can be deduced that students at the School of Midwifery run a high percentage of risks, especially female students, for diseases or problems related to cardiovascular disorders, colon disorders, academic problems, suicide, unwanted pregnancies, infectious diseases, violence, and mental health problems.

Finally, by analysing each dimension, it can be understood that lifestyle is the set of behavioural habits that constitute protective factors for health or risk factors for disease, taking into account the way of life and living conditions12.

In the present research, healthy lifestyles in the students of the School of Obstetrics predominate in the dimensions of physical activity and eating habits with 70% and 60%; likewise, unhealthy lifestyles predominate in the dimensions of sleep-stress and consumption of toxic substances with 70% and 80%. These data differ from the study by Campo et al, carried out in a Higher Education Institution in Bogotá called Healthy lifestyles and risk behaviours in medical students, in which it was concluded that there is a healthy lifestyle in most of the dimensions evaluated among medical students8.

It is evident that in the students of the School of Obstetrics, the unhealthy lifestyle tips the balance in their favour, this brings with it various risks, according to the dimensions where it has been most evident; this would diminish their capacities and plans in the professional field, with their patients, mostly pregnant women, being indirectly affected in the future.

CHAPTER VI

CONCLUSIONS:

The results of this research lead to the following conclusions:

1. Most of the students of the School of Midwifery in the dimension of physical activity do physical exercise, with a frequency and time considered adequate; nevertheless, a percentage of sedentary lifestyle persists, which would expose them to the risk of various cardiovascular and non-communicable diseases.

2. In the dietary habits dimension, a good percentage of the population studied showed adequate eating habits, thanks to a good quantity of liquid intake, as well as a considerable consumption of foods containing saturated fats, sugars and salt, in addition to a much lower intake of fruit, nuts, vegetables, pulses and cereals than recommended.

3. In the sleep and stress dimension, a high percentage of university students were identified who reported having symptoms of stress and who consider academic overload to be the situation that causes them most stress, which shows a high degree of affectation in the short and long term mental health of the population under study.

4. In the dimension of consumption of toxic substances, a high percentage of students showed an inclination towards the consumption of cigarettes and alcohol, while another group reported having occasionally consumed some type of drugs; these situations could influence their academic performance, altering their psycho-emotional state (mental health), and indirectly affecting the health of their future patients to whom they will provide health services, in this case pregnant women.

CHAPTER VII

RECOMMENDATIONS:

1. It is recommended that the management of the School of Obstetrics, in coordination with the area of university welfare of the National University of Tumbes, strengthen the activities that promote daily physical activity, which should be mostly aerobic, this in the framework of the "global recommendations on physical activity for health" given by the WHO in 2010.

2. It is recommended that the management of the School of Nutrition, through the area of university welfare, encourage the creation of food systems that promote a diversified, balanced diet in the different canteens located within the central university campus, as well as in the headquarters of the different faculties of the National University of Tumbes.

3. It is recommended that the management, in coordination with the head of the department of the School of Midwifery, convene regular meetings to evaluate the implementation of an individual programme for stress management and sleep reconciliation, taking into account the aspects that contribute to its treatment, such as physical activity, nutrition and social support, improving academic schedules and optimising personalised tutoring.

4. It is recommended that within the tutoring programme, students with a history of substance abuse and low academic performance should work closely with a psychologist, and that awareness campaigns should be carried out to raise awareness of the damage to health caused by cigarettes and alcohol, so that the students of the School of Midwifery do not suffer the long-term consequences of the consumption of these products.

CHAPTER

VIII BIBLIOGRAPHICAL REFERENCES

1.   González J, Cuevas R. Physical activity as a model of health promotion, individual adaptation and healthy effort in adolescence. EFDeportes.com, Digital Magazine. [Internet]. Buenos Aires 2015 [citado 07 enerode2018   ]

   20(204):1-1.from: http://www.efdeportes.com/efd204/actividad-fisica-esfuerzo-saludable- en-la-adolescencia.htm

2.   Sánchez M, Luna E. Healthy lifestyle habits in the university population. Nutr Hosp [Internet]. Spain 2014 [cited 07 January 2018] 31(5):1910 -1919. DOI:10.3305/nh.2015.31.5.8608

3.   Ministry of Education, Culture and Sport (MECD). Lifestyles and health of university students [blog on the Internet]. Madrid (Spain): MECD. May 2015 [cited 07 January 2018] retrieved from: http://blogbibliotecas.mecd.gob.es/2015/05/20/ estilos-de-vida-y-salud-des-los-universitarios/

4.   Bennasar M. Lifestyles and health in university students, [Doctoral thesis]. Illes Balears: publication centre of the University of Illes Balears; Spain, 2011 [cited 05 November 2017]. Retrieved from: http://www.tdx.cat/handle/10803/84136

5.   Trujillo J, Wilman P. Sleep and time allocation among university students: the case of the Universidad del Atlántico. Semestre Económico; Colombia 2010 13(27), 99-116 [cited 05 November 2017]. Retrieved from: http://www.scielo.org.co/pdf/seec/v13n27 /v13n27a6.pdf

6. Ratner G, Hernández J, Martel A, Atalah S. Food quality and nutritional status in university students from 11 regions of Chile. Rev. Méd. Chile [Internet]. 2012 140(12): 1571-1579. [cited 2017 Nov 05]. DOI: 10.4067/S0034-98872012001200008

7. Becerra F, Pinzón G, Vargas M. Nutritional status and food consumption of university students admitted to the career of Medicine. Bogotá 2010-2011. Rev. Fac. Med. Colombia 2012; 60 (Suppl): S3-12. [cited 2017 Nov 05]. Retrieved from: http://www.bdigital.unal.edu.co/35216/1/35472-139226-1-PB.pdf

8. Campo Y, Pombo LM, Teherán A. Healthy lifestyles and risk behaviours in medical students. Rev. Univ. Ind. Santander. Health [Internet]. Colombia 2016 Sep. 48(3): 301-309 [cited 2017 Nov 03]. DOI: 10.18273/revsal.v48n3-2016004

9. Tamayo J, Rodríguez K, Escobar K, Mejía A. Lifestyles of dental students. Hacia promoc. salud. Colombia 2015 20(2): 147-160 [cited 04 November 2017]. DOI:10.17151/ hpsal.2015.20.2.10

10. Atucha N, Cecilia J. and Garcia J. Health styles and healthy habits in students of the Degree in Pharmacy. Educ Med. 2017 [cited 2017 Nov 06]. DOI: https://doi.org/10.1016/j.edumed.2017.07.008

11. Barrenechea L, Gómez Z, Huaira P, Pregúntegui L, Aguirre G, Rey de C. Sleep quality and excessive daytime sleepiness in third and fourth year medical students. CIMEL Latin American Student Medical Science and Research [Internet]. Peru 2010;15(2):54-58 [cited 2017 Nov 06]. Retrieved from: http://www.redalyc.org /articulo.oa?id=71721155002

12. Becerra S. Role of perceived stress and its coping in the health behaviors of university students in Lima [Tesis Magistral]. Lima: Repositorio Digital de Tesis PUCP, revista Psicología Clínica de la Salud, Pontificia Universidad Católica del Perú; 2013 [cited 2017 Nov 06]. Retrieved from: http://tesis.pucp.edu.pe/repositorio /handle/123456789/5013

13. Vílchez J., Quiñones D., Failoc V., Acevedo T., Larico G., Mucching S. et al. Mental health and sleep quality in students from eight human medical schools in Peru. Rev. chil. neuro-psychiatr. [internet]. 2016 54(4): 272-281. [cited 2017 Nov 06]. DOI: http://dx.doi.org/10.4067/S0717-92272016000400002.

14. Beltrán C. Estilo de vida en jóvenes universitarios de la facultad de psicología de la fundación universitaria de los libertadores, [Tesis de grado]. Bogotá: digital repository fundación universitaria Los Libertadores; Colombia, 2016 [cited 2017 Nov 07]. Retrieved from: http://repository.libertadores.edu.co/bitstream/ handle/11371/958/Beltr%C3%A1nCorredorMarily.pdf?sequence=2

15. Varela MT, Duarte C, Salazar IC, Lema LF. Physical activity and sedentary lifestyle in young university students in Colombia: practices, motives and resources to perform them. Colomb Med 2011 42(3): 269-77. [cited 2017 Nov 06]. Retrieved from: http://www.bioline.org.b r/pdf?rc11049

16. Vidarte J, Vélez C., Sandoval C., Mora M. Physical activity: health promotion strategy, Hacia la Promoción de la Salud journal, Colombia 2011 [cited February 09, 2018] 16(1):202-218. Retrieved from: http://www.scielo.org.co/pdf/hpsal/v16n1/v16n 1a14.pdf

17. Fernanda M, Oviedo G. Lifestyles, motivations, resources and cardiovascular risk in nursing students. [Degree thesis]. Cali: Universidad del Valle Digital Library, Universidad del Valle; 2013 [cited 2017 Nov 10]. Retrieved from: http://bibliotecadigital.univalle.edu.co/xmlui/bitstream/handle/10893/9574/ CB-0516592.pdf?sequence=1

18. Carina P. Nutritional status and eating habits in fourth year students of the Bachelor's Degree in Nutrition. [Tesis Licenciatura], Universidad Abierta Interamericana de Argentina; 2012 [cited 2017 November 11]. Retrieved from: http://imgbiblio.vaneduc.edu.ar/ fulltext/files/TC111967.pdf

19. Vílchez C, Quiñones L, Failoc R, Acevedo V, Larico C, Mucching T, et al. Mental health and sleep quality in students from eight human medical schools in Peru. Rev. chil. neuro-psychiatr. [Internet]. 2016; 54(4): 272-281 [cited 2017 Nov 06]. DOI: 10.4067/S0717- 92272016000400002.

20. Martín M. Academic stress in university students. Apuntes de Psicología. Spain 2007 25(1): 87-99 [cited 2017 Nov 05]. Retrieved from: http://www.apuntesdepsicologia.es/index.php/ revista/article/view/117

21. Cano A. The nature of stress [Internet]. Spain: Spanish Society for the study of anxiety and stress [cited 2017 Nov 06]. Retrieved from: http://webs.ucm.es/info/ seas/estres_lab/el_estres.htm.

22. Segura O, Aguilar M, Fajardo A. Characterization of healthy lifestyles in undergraduate students of the Faculty of Medical Sciences of the University of San Carlos de Guatemala April-July 2014. [Tesis Licenciatura], Universidad de San Carlos de Guatemala [cited 2017 Nov 07]. Retrieved from: http://www.repositorio.usac.edu.gt/id/eprint/704

23. Díaz B, Maca M, Melo M, Rico V. Characteristics of lifestyles in students of the san buenaventura university Bogotá campus. [Tesis Licenciatura], Universidad de San Buenaventura de Bogotá [cited 2017 Nov 07]. Retrieved from: http://biblioteca.usbbog.edu.co:8080/Biblioteca/BDigital/BDigital/83524.pdf

24. Muñoz G, Aguilera A. El consumo de sustancias nocivas a la salud en estudiantes de primaria y secundaria. In: Paper presented at the IX Congreso Nacional de Investigación Educativa. Yucatán: Consejo Mexicano de Investigación Educativa, A.C; 2007. p.1-12. [cited 07 November 2017]. Retrieved from: http://www.comie.org.mx/congreso/memoriaelectronica/v09/ponencias/at06/PRE1178936433.pdf

25. Osorio J. Ethical principles of human and animal research. MEDICINA (Buenos Aires) 2000; 60: 255-258 [cited 2017 Nov 05]. Retrieved from: http://www.medicinabuenosaires.com/demo/revistas/vol60-00/2/v60_n2_255_258.pdf

26. Irazusta A, Ruiz F, Gil S, Gil FJ, Irazusta J. Lifestyle habits of nursing students. Zainak [journal on the Internet] 2005 [cited 07 January 2018]; 27:99-107. Retrieved from: http://hedatuz.euskomedia.org/3806/1/27099107.pdf

Table of Contents

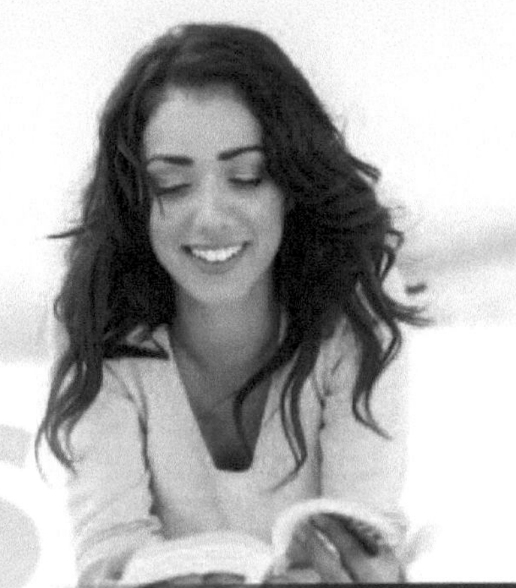

yes
I want morebooks!

Buy your books fast and straightforward online - at one of world's fastest growing online book stores! Environmentally sound due to Print-on-Demand technologies.

Buy your books online at
www.morebooks.shop

Kaufen Sie Ihre Bücher schnell und unkompliziert online – auf einer der am schnellsten wachsenden Buchhandelsplattformen weltweit! Dank Print-On-Demand umwelt- und ressourcenschonend produzi ert.

Bücher schneller online kaufen
www.morebooks.shop

KS OmniScriptum Publishing
Brivibas gatve 197
LV-1039 Riga, Latvia
Telefax: +371 686 204 55

info@omniscriptum.com
www.omniscriptum.com

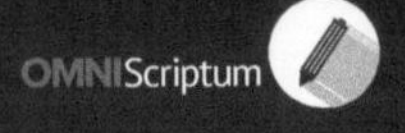

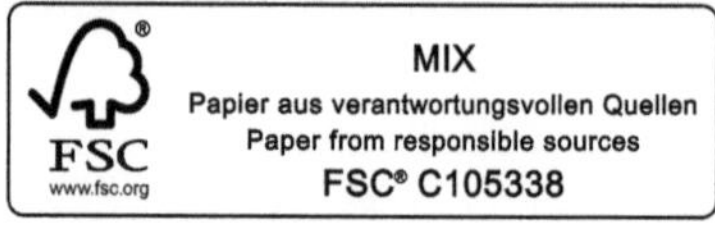

Printed by Books on Demand GmbH, Norderstedt / Germany